Journal for An Invitation to Personal Change

Dianne Hales, M.S. | Kenneth W. Christian, Ph.D.

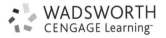

WADSWORTH
CENGAGE Learning

Australia • Brazil • Japan • Korea • Mexico • Singapore • Spain • United Kingdom • United States

WADSWORTH
CENGAGE Learning™

Journal for An Invitation to Personal Change
Dianne Hales, Kenneth W. Christian

Development Editor: Anna Lustig

Assistant Editor: Elesha Feldman

Editorial Assistant: Sarah Farrant

Technology Project Manager: Lauren Tarson

Marketing Assistant: Katherine Malatesta

Marketing Communications Manager:
  Belinda Krohmer

Project Manager, Editorial Production:
  Trudy Brown

Creative Director: Rob Hugel

Art Director: John Walker

Print Buyer: Paula Vang

Permissions Editor: Bob Kauser

Production Service: Graphic World Inc.

Text Designer: Jeanne Calabrese

Cover Designer: Bill Stanton

Cover Image: Beth Dixson/Alamy

Compositor: Graphic World Inc.

For product information and technology assistance, contact us at
Cengage Learning Customer & Sales Support, 1-800-354-9706
For permission to use material from this text or product,
submit all requests online at **cengage.com/permissions**
Further permissions questions can be e-mailed to
permissionrequest@cengage.com

Library of Congress Control Number: 2008923822

ISBN-13: 978-0-495-55710-4

ISBN-10: 0-495-55710-2

Wadsworth
10 Davis Drive
Belmont, CA 94002-3098
USA

Cengage Learning is a leading provider of customized learning solutions with office locations around the globe, including Singapore, the United Kingdom, Australia, Mexico, Brazil, and Japan. Locate your local office at **international.cengage.com/region**

Cengage Learning products are represented in Canada by Nelson Education, Ltd.

For your course and learning solutions, visit **academic.cengage.com**

Purchase any of our products at your local college store or at our preferred online store **www.ichapters.com**

Printed in Canada
1 2 3 4 5 6 7 12 11 10 09 08

CONTENTS

INTRODUCTION

The book you hold in your hands is different from any other book you are likely to use for a college class. Although you will find inspirational content and instructions for exercises and iChange labs, ultimately you will become the author of this book. As we point out in *An Invitation to Personal Change* (IPC), you write your own life story by the changes you make every day. When you change your choices, you change your story. This journal shows you how to do this—step by step and exercise by exercise.

Maybe you already write regularly in a journal and have done so for a long time. If so, you already know the benefits that come from recording your personal thoughts and reflections. If not, you are about to discover a power tool for knowing yourself more intimately and for directing personal change.

Your *Journal for An Invitation to Personal Change,* as you will quickly see, is a tightly integrated companion to IPC. Each exercise in the book has a place devoted to it here in the *IPC Journal* in the same order in which it appears in IPC and is clearly labeled and cross-referenced to the text. For each of the many journal entries assigned in IPC, you will find appropriate space for structured self-ratings and more open-ended observations and reflections.

Your *IPC Journal* is a valuable tool for conveniently keeping all your work in one place. Moreover, by using a journal expressly designed for use with IPC, you will work efficiently and enjoy the assignments more fully.

Nevertheless, we have a broader, unhidden agenda: to introduce and extend your appreciation of journaling as a lifelong personal change tool. Take advantage of its power, its rewards—and its unlimited potential for enhancing your personal growth and your life.

The following sections correspond to the material in *An Invitation to Personal Change.*

Chapter 4: Your Personal GPS

Start by asking yourself three key questions:

1. What am I doing now that I want to stop doing?

_____

_____

_____

_____

_____

_____

2. What am I *not* doing now that I want to do?

_____

_____

_____

_____

_____

_____

3. What am I doing now that I want to increase or decrease?

_____

_____

_____

_____

_____

_____

Assess Yourself

1. Write down a number from 0 to 100 for how you usually feel about yourself. Let 0 represent the worst you could possibly feel about yourself and 100 the best you could possibly feel about yourself.

    _____

    Circle this number. It stands for how you *usually* feel about yourself.

2. Write down a second number from 0 to 100 for how you feel about yourself *now*. Put the current date beside this number.

    _____   _____

3. List the qualities that make you feel good about yourself as a person.

    _____

    _____

    _____

    _____

    _____

    _____

    _____

    _____

    _____

    _____

    _____

4. List the qualities that make you feel badly about yourself as a person.

    _____

    _____

    _____

    _____

    _____

    _____

    _____

    _____

    _____

    _____

    _____

5. Write down major assets (such as life experience, a supportive family, special talents, experience living in foreign cultures, or a second or even third language) that you have not yet listed.

_____

_____

_____

_____

_____

_____

_____

_____

6. Write down what you consider to be your major limitations (such as financial problems, disabilities, or cultural barriers) that you haven't yet listed.

_____

_____

_____

_____

_____

_____

_____

_____

Create a Timeline

Get a large, poster-sized sheet of paper. On the top half, construct a timeline of your life with an arbitrary life span of 90 years. Mark the events of your life up to the present moment, noting major milestones.

Mark the spot on your timeline that represents today. Based on your self-appraisal and the change you have in mind, mark the date by which you think you will be ready to make your desired change. Look at your timeline and pencil in the major steps you need to take each day, week, or month to make your desired change.

Chapter 5: Call for Order

One Change at a Time

Identify one problem or hassle caused by a lack of order in your life. Describe the consequences of this specific form of disorder. Then think of one simple change you could make that would prevent or correct it. Try out your solution for three weeks. If you don't see a significant difference, reflect on what you have learned during the three weeks and come up with a more effective modification.

_____

_____

_____

_____

_____

Chapter 6: Time Control

Build Pleasure into Your Day

1. Record how you spend your time over a period that includes at least one weekend day. Put a plus sign next to those activities that energized or excited you and a minus sign next to those that drained you.

2. Identify positive practices you can weave into your daily routine, such as listening to a playlist of music that stirs or soothes you or looking at the night sky.

_____

_____

_____

_____

_____

Practice Real-Time Writing

As soon as you read through this assignment, start writing in the space that follows. Describe your typical attitude and approach to writing.

_____

_____

_____

_____

_____

_____

_____

_____

_____

_____

_____

_____

_____

_____

_____

_____

_____

_____

_____

_____

_____

_____

_____

_____

_____

_____

_____

Chapter 7: Learning the Language of Change

No More Negatives

Make a list of some positive attributes you plan to acquire. For example, if you'd like to be assertive, confident, and self-assured, claim these characteristics as your own now.

_____

_____

_____

_____

_____

Write a series of statements describing the new, improved you—all in the present tense.

_____

_____

_____

_____

_____

_____

What Do You Choose?

1. Go back to the list of negative or limiting attributes you compiled in your journal entries for Chapter 4. Take five of these characteristics and, in the space at the end of these instructions, make a simple, self-descriptive statement with each one. For example, if you listed "procrastination," you might write, "I am a procrastinator."

_____

_____

_____

_____

_____

2. Now write a sentence that gives an example or description of each behavior.

_____

_____

_____

_____

_____

3. Next, rewrite each sentence, inserting the word _choose_.

_____

_____

_____

_____

_____

4. Now rewrite each sentence again, making the following significant change: Put the sentence in the past tense and modify it with an adverb, like _often_, that acknowledges you have not always behaved in the same way.

_____

_____

_____

_____

_____

5. When you have completed the preceding steps, reread all forms of the sentences you have written, noticing the difference each simple change makes in the way you experience choice and the possibility for change.

6. Now take this exercise to a new level: In the space that follows, write a sentence about each new positive behavior.

_____

_____

_____

_____

_____

7. After you complete the new positive alternative sentence, take another long look at the sentences you have written about each behavior. Let the progression sink in.

8. For two full weeks, repeat the new final sentence you have written five times upon rising and five times before sleeping.

Just Because

Write new sentences describing your behavior, using the following pattern:

I _____ because _____.

I _____ because _____.

I _____ because _____.

I _____ because _____.

I _____ because _____.

Chapter 8: Going for Your Goals

Dream Big

If you already know your dream, write it here.

_____

_____

_____

_____

_____

_____

_____

_____

_____

_____

_____

_____

_____

If you do not have a specific dream or vision yet, write down your vision, your big-picture dream, and your wildest, most outrageous, even your most far-fetched hopes and goals.

_____

_____

_____

_____

_____

_____

_____

_____

_____

_____

_____

_____

Now write answers to the following questions. Write quickly, allowing no more than 60 to 90 seconds for every answer. If an answer doesn't come to you in that time, skip the question and move on to the next one.

1. What do you want your life to be like?

_____

_____

_____

_____

2. What draws your attention and taps into your enthusiasm? What fascinates you, intrigues you, or tickles your curiosity?

_____

_____

_____

_____

_____

_____

3. What would you do if you were guaranteed 100 percent success?

_____

_____

_____

_____

_____

_____

4. If you had the self-esteem necessary to be unstoppable, what would you do differently?

_____

_____

_____

_____

_____

5. As a child, what did you first seriously imagine you would do when you grew up? What was your first true ambition?

_____

_____

_____

_____

_____

6. What qualities continue to inspire respect and awe in you? What qualities would you develop in yourself if you knew how?

_____

_____

_____

_____

_____

_____

7. What would you plan to do in the future if you didn't have to earn money to make a living?

_____

_____

_____

_____

_____

_____

Look at these questions daily and keep answering them until you hit pay dirt or run out of new things to say. If you can answer all of them the first day, fine. If you draw a blank on one or more of them, take another look the next day and see what comes to you. If after a week you can't come up with one specific dream, in the space that follows list the things you want to do, experience, or master before you die. Choose one idea from this list to use as your vision as you continue working through this chapter.

_____

_____

_____

_____

_____

_____

Setting Long-Term Goals

1. Review your descriptions of your dreams and visions, and translate them into one overarching dream and a handful of specific, long-term goals.
2. Turn your vision into a goal. Setting goals in the right way increases their effectiveness, so write your long-term goals in the present tense as if you've already achieved them.

3. Write no more than five or six long-term goals in this fashion.

_____

_____

_____

_____

_____

_____

4. Do not set a time limit for these goals.
5. Repeat each goal five times in the morning and five times at night until you reach it. This exercise makes your long-term goal function as a command directing you to make efforts toward meeting it.

Chapter 9: Power Journaling

Jump-Start Your Journaling

To get going, complete one of the following sentences:

1. When I think about my life, I wish I had _____

_____

_____

_____

_____

2. When I reflect on my habits, they seem _____

_____

_____

_____

_____

3. Thinking about the way I handle relationships, I feel _____

_____

_____

_____

_____

Journaling for Better Health and Wellness

Once you've identified a target health goal, write it in the space that follows.

_____

_____

_____

Now do the following exercise:

1. Identify your best health habits. Write down everything you are doing to improve your health and wellness.

_____

_____

_____

_____

_____

_____

_____

_____

_____

2. Honestly list your worst health habits. Write down what you are doing that is not good for your body, mind, or spirit.

_____

_____

_____

_____

_____

_____

_____

_____

_____

3. Ask yourself and answer in writing: What is one thing I could do to improve my health and enhance my wellness?

_____

_____

_____

4. Ask yourself: What could I do right away?

_____

_____

_____

5. Today?

_____

_____

_____

6. This week?

_____

_____

_____

7. This month?

_____

_____

_____

8. Write down one thing that you will do, as soon as possible, to improve your health.

_____

_____

_____

Letters You Never Send

Write a letter to a person, place, event, even an attitude. Begin with a salutation, just as you would if you were writing a letter: "Dear...." Then let your pen lead you. Afterward, if you want to do more with what you've written, share it with a trusted friend or counselor.

_____

_____

_____

_____

_____

_____

_____

_____

_____

Chapter 10: Making Yourself Lucky

Making It Real

Practice your new behaviors in real life. Each day create as many opportunities as possible in which to use your new instructions, including simulations. In the space that follows, keep track of how often you follow your new operating instructions. Notice how quickly they become automatic.

_____

_____

_____

_____

_____

Chapter 11: Reaching Out

Whom Do You Need?

1. Spend some time considering the type of support you could best use and whom you could enlist to accompany you while you change. Make a list of your needs and wishes and the qualities you think would help you most.

_____

_____

_____

_____

_____

_____

_____

_____

_____

_____

_____

2. Jot down the names of potential candidates, and audition them in your mind.

_____

_____

_____

_____

_____

_____

_____

_____

_____

_____

_____

_____

Log on for Virtual Support

Search the Internet for websites related to the behaviors you want to change or the habits you wish to create. Make a list of the most useful sites, which might include blogs, bulletin boards, chat groups, and web pages created by professional organizations or commercial sponsors.

_____

_____

_____

_____

_____

_____

Chapter 12: Shock Absorption

Check Your GPS: Where Are You Now?

If you know or suspect you may have drifted, check your bearings. Go back to entries earlier in this journal for Chapter 4, read what you wrote, and then ask yourself the following questions:

1. Where were you intending to go when you started out?

_____

_____

_____

_____

_____

2. What was your aim?

_____

_____

_____

_____

_____

_____

3. Is it still the same?

_____

_____

_____

_____

_____

"If you continue on the path you are on," a Chinese aphorism states, "you will get to where you are going." If this notion distresses you, you may have strayed from your path. If it fills you with relief and reassurance, you are likely still headed in the right direction. If your reactions are mixed, ask yourself again the questions we first posed in Chapter 4, "Your Personal GPS":

1. What am I doing now that I want to stop doing?

_____

_____

_____

_____

_____

2. What am I *not* doing now that I want to do?

_____

_____

_____

_____

_____

3. What am I doing now that I want to increase or decrease?

_____

_____

_____

_____

_____

_____

Your Best Mistake

Describe a mistake you made or setback you've experienced in the space that follows. Then note what you learned from handling this setback, what strengths and strategies helped you through it, what you adjusted, and how much stronger you are for overcoming it.

_____

_____

_____

_____

_____

_____

_____

_____

Whose Goals Are You Pursuing?

List each change goal you have created. For each one, examine the source and inspiration for the particular goal. (There is nothing wrong if the inspiration came from someone other than you.)

Give each goal a rating from 0 to 100 for the degree to which the goal is one you embrace as your own, using 0 for one that you do not embrace and 100 for a goal fully embraced by you. Make a second rating to express the importance of accomplishing each goal, using 0 for a goal completely unimportant to you and 100 for one as important as you could imagine.

_____ _____ _____

_____ _____ _____

_____ _____ _____

_____ _____ _____

_____ _____ _____

_____ _____ _____

Now make some additional notes about what you have learned from this journaling exercise.

_____

_____

_____

_____

_____

_____

_____

_____

The following exercises correspond to the content in *Labs for An Invitation to Personal Change.*

Lab 1: Choosing to Change, Choosing a Change

Get Real

In order to choose a change, start by appraising where you are now in relation to making a choice.

1. HOW CLOSE ARE YOU TO MAKING A CHOICE?

In the space that follows, write a number from 0 to 100 to describe how close, or ready, you are to making a choice, with 0 representing that you are not ready and 100 representing that you are completely ready to choose.

_____

2. WHAT IS YOUR USUAL APPROACH TO CHOOSING?

Observe how you make choices now, and survey how you have made choices in the past.

Respond to each of the following questions. Be honest. You have no one to fool. Do not show your answers to anyone else.

▪ Do you usually avoid choosing?

_____

_____

_____

▪ Would you ordinarily look for what would appear to be the easiest lab to knock out without any effort?

_____

_____

_____

■ Are you afraid to choose because you feel you could choose incorrectly?

_____

_____

_____

■ Do you wonder what you "should" choose, in the sense of what others will think?

_____

_____

_____

3. HOW DO YOU FEEL ABOUT CHOOSING A LAB?

Answer the following:

■ Does picking a particular lab feel like admitting weakness?
■ Is there anything you are afraid to admit?
■ Are you avoiding a change you might like to make because you are afraid you might fail?
■ Do the changes suggested by the labs feel too big to tackle?

4. GO FOR QUALITY.

Read the following two paragraphs and write your response to the question that follows them:

Whether or not you are using these labs for a class, we suggest that you take on no more than two labs at a time. In addition to completing this lab, we recommend that you choose no more than one other lab to do now. But if you feel more ambitious, keep to a maximum of no more than two other labs that you complete simultaneously.

Why not try more? One good experience that you truly savor is far more worthwhile than four or five labs done merely for extra credit or to pad your grade. This book is about more than a grade and more than just meeting a class requirement. It is about your life and how you live it. The way you approach the labs is not isolated from the way you live the rest of your life. Go for quality. Get real about this.

Respond to this question: Do I go for quality?

_____

_____

_____

_____

_____

_____

_____

5. TRACK YOUR CHOICES.

For three consecutive days, record five choices you make during each day.

1. _____ _____

2. _____ _____

3. _____ _____

4. _____ _____

5. _____ _____

Note beside each choice whether you chose in favor of quality, quantity, speed, or just to get something out of the way.

6. EVALUATE PAST DECISIONS.

List five important decisions you have made in your life to date. Record the following for each one:

▪ How the decision turned out
▪ Whether you consulted anyone for advice and, if so, whom
▪ Your appraisal of the benefits of the decision
▪ Your appraisal of any drawbacks of the decision

1.

_____

_____

_____

_____

_____

_____

2.

_____

_____

_____

_____

_____

_____

_____

3.

_____

_____

_____

_____

_____

4.

_____

_____

_____

_____

_____

5.

_____

_____

_____

_____

_____

Get Ready

1. ASSESS YOUR GREATEST CHANGE NEEDS.

Most people know some areas they need to change. For you it could be order, diet, exercise, or finding balance in your life. In the spaces that follow, list the changes you would like to make if only you knew how. Then rate which one is the most pressing, most important need to deal with first.

_____   _____

_____   _____

_____   _____

_____   _____

2. CHECK OUT THE AVAILABLE LABS.

To get a better feel for the possibilities they present, read at least the introduction of each lab. This is the section before "Get Real." After reading each introduction, use a five-point scale (with 0 as no interest and 5 as highest) to rate your interest in making the particular change. Do this in two ways:

■ Rate how appealing this lab would be to do *at some point.*

■ Rate how valuable you feel this lab would be to do *now.*

Lab 2.	The Grateful Thread	_____	_____
Lab 3.	Soul Food	_____	_____
Lab 4.	Your Personal Balance Point	_____	_____
Lab 5.	Defusing Test Stress	_____	_____
Lab 6.	Rx: Relax	_____	_____
Lab 7.	Do It Now	_____	_____
Lab 8.	Your Psychological Self-Care Pyramid	_____	_____
Lab 9.	Help Yourself	_____	_____
Lab 10.	Excise Exercise Excuses	_____	_____
Lab 11.	Mind over Platter	_____	_____
Lab 12.	Thinking Thinner	_____	_____
Lab 13.	Listen Up	_____	_____
Lab 14.	What's Your Intimacy Quotient?	_____	_____
Lab 15.	To Have or Have Not	_____	_____
Lab 16.	Don't Go There	_____	_____
Lab 17.	Your Alcohol Audit	_____	_____
Lab 18.	Butt Out	_____	_____
Lab 19.	Taming a Toxic Temper	_____	_____
Lab 20.	Sleep Power	_____	_____
Lab 21.	The Sexiness of Safer Sex	_____	_____
Lab 22.	Health Assurance	_____	_____
Lab 23.	Your Guardian Angel	_____	_____
Lab 24.	OurSpace	_____	_____
Lab 25.	Finity	_____	_____

Add the two numbers you assigned to the labs. Did you give any of them two fives? Which labs gained the highest scores?

_____

_____

_____

_____

3. SEE WHICH OF THE HIGHEST-SCORING LABS CORRESPOND BEST TO YOUR PRIME NEEDS FOR CHANGE.

Take a look at the list you created of your greatest change needs. Now see how well the list of favored labs compares to your greatest change needs. You may see an obvious choice for the lab to do.

If you do not see one clear choice, appraise anything else you need to know, or do, in order to be ready to choose. Make a journal entry describing what you need to know and do.

4. APPRAISE ANYTHING ELSE YOU NEED TO KNOW, OR DO, IN ORDER TO BE READY TO CHOOSE.

Make a journal entry describing what you need to know and do.

_____

_____

_____

_____

_____

_____

_____

_____

_____

_____

_____

When you have completed that entry, do whatever you need to do.

In the end, make the best choice you can. Do not get caught up in obsessing about whether your choice is perfect. Remember, you can do every lab in the book at some time. Just select one to do now.

Get Going

Your next task is straightforward: *Get started working on your goal*.

Turn to the page where the lab begins. Take the primary steps outlined in the "Get Real" section now.

Lock It In

Once you decide on a change, lock it in by reporting your choice to your accountability partner. If you are taking a class, your instructor may serve this role.

Stay with the lab you chose. You may hit flat spots of disinterest. Even if you become discouraged, however, we strongly urge you to keep going. Do not entertain for a second the notion that you chose poorly or that you should start over on another lab.

Good luck and enjoy the voyage!

What follows next in your journal is space set aside for you to complete the journaling requested for six labs you choose to complete. You will find space available at the beginning of each section to write the Lab number and Lab title and then room to record your thoughts and responses to questions under the "Get Real," "Get Ready," "Get Going," and "Lock It In" headings. Finally, we add a page in each section (you may need more) for your iChange report.

As we have said before, this is the template for every lab in IPC and one you can use for any future labs you wish to complete or any other behavior change you wish to make.

GET REAL

_____

_____

_____

_____

"It's not that some people have will-power and some don't. It's that some people are ready to change and others are not."

–James Gordon, M.D.

_____

_____

_____

_____

_____

_____

_____

_____

_____

_____

_____

_____

_____

_____

_____

_____

_____

_____

_____

_____

_____

_____

_____

_____

_____

_____

_____   *"If we go down
into ourselves,
we find that we
possess exactly
what we desire."*

—Simone Weil

_____

_____

_____

_____

_____

_____

_____

29

_____

_____

_____

_____

_____

_____

_____

_____

_____

"Treat people as if they were what they ought to be and you will help them become what they are capable of becoming."

–Johann Wolfgang von Goethe

GET READY

_____

_____

_____

_____

_____

_____

_____   *"My failed paintings
                                 teach me to go in
_____   another direction.
                                 My ordinary paint-
_____   ings teach me my
                                 craft. My extraordi-
_____   nary paintings
                                 teach me to aspire
_____   to a higher level of
                                 achievement."*

_____   —Ellen McCormick Martens

_____

_____   33

_____

_____

_____

_____

_____

_____

_____

_____

_____

_____

_____

_____

_____

> *"Just remember the world is not a playground but a schoolroom. Life is not a holiday but an education. One eternal lesson for us all: to teach us how better we should love."*
>
> –Barbara Jordan

GET GOING

"A man who views the world the same at fifty as he did at twenty has wasted thirty years of his life."

—Muhammad Ali

_____

_____

_____

_____

_____

_____

_____

_____

_____

"I hated every minute of training, but I said, 'Don't quit. Suffer now and live the rest of your life as a champion.'"

–Muhammad Ali

_____

_____

_____

_____

_____

_____

_____

_____

_____

_____

_____

_____

_____

_____

_____

_____

"The soul becomes dyed with the colors of its thoughts."

–Marcus Aurelius

LOCK IT IN

*"There are
treasures hidden in
the human mind."*

–Sarane Alexandrian

> *"We write to taste life twice, in the moment and in retrospection."*
>
> –Anais Nin

42

İCHANGE REPORT

_____

_____

_____

_____

_____

_____

"Live for yourself and you will live in vain. Live for others and you will live again."

—Peter Tosh

_____

_____

_____

_____

_____

_____

_____

44

_____

_____

_____

_____

_____

_____

_____

_____

_____

_____

_____

Lab number: _____ Name of Lab: _____

GET REAL

_____

_____

_____

_____

_____

_____

_____

_____

_____

_____

"The best and most beautiful things in the world cannot be seen or even touched. They must be felt with the heart."

–Helen Keller

_____

_____

_____

_____

_____

_____

_____

_____

_____

_____

_____

_____

_____

_____

_____

_____

_____

"Life begets life. Energy creates energy. It is by spending oneself that one becomes rich."

−Sarah Bernhardt

_____

_____

_____

_____ *"The giving of love*
is an education in
_____ *itself."*

_____ —Eleanor Roosevelt

_____

_____

_____

_____

_____

_____

_____

_____

_____

_____

_____

_____

_____

_____

_____

_____

_____

_____

GET READY

---

*"There are no
limits, just edges."*

–Jackson Pollock

51

GET GOING

_____

_____

_____

_____

_____

_____

*"You should be the
one to kick the rock
off the road."*

–Gabriela Mistral

_____

_____

_____

_____

_____

_____

_____

_____

_____

_____

_____

_____

_____

_____

_____

_____

_____

_____

_____

> *"Life is denied by lack of attention, whether it be to cleaning windows or trying to write a masterpiece."*
>
> —Nadia Boulanger

LOCK IT IN

_____

_____

_____

_____

_____

_____

_____

_____

> *"Knowing others is intelligence; knowing yourself is true wisdom. Mastering others is strength; mastering yourself is true power."*
>
> —Lao Tzu

_____

_____

_____

_____

_____

_____

_____

_____

_____

_____

_____

_____

_____

_____

_____

*"If there were
dreams to sell,
What would
you buy?"*
—Thomas Lovell Beddoes

iCHANGE REPORT

_____

_____

_____

_____ *"Most people are*
about as happy as
_____ *they make up their*
minds to be."
_____ –Abraham Lincoln

_____

_____

_____

_____

_____

_____

_____

_____

_____

_____

_____

_____

_____

_____

_____

_____

GET REAL

_____

_____

_____

_____

_____

_____

_____

_____

"Let us be grateful to people who make us happy; they are the charming gardeners who make our souls blossom."

–Marcel Proust

_____

_____

_____

_____

_____

_____

_____

_____

_____

_____

_____

_____

_____

_____

_____

_____

_____

_____

_____

_____

_____

_____

_____

_____

_____

_____   *"Permanence,*
perseverance, and
_____   *persistence in spite*
of all obstacles,
_____   *discouragements,*
and impossibilities:
_____   *it is this in all things*
that distinguishes
_____   *the strong soul from*
the weak."

–Thomas Carlyle

_____

_____   63

_____

_____

_____

_____

_____

_____

_____

_____

_____

GET READY

> *"Work is the grand cure of all the maladies and miseries that ever beset mankind."*
>
> –Thomas Carlyle

_____

_____

_____

_____

_____

_____

_____

_____

_____

_____

_____

_____

_____

_____

_____

_____

_____

_____

_____

_____

_____

_____

_____

_____

_____

"If we had no winter, the spring would not be so pleasant; if we did not sometimes taste adversity, prosperity would not be so welcome."

—Anne Bradstreet

GET GOING

> *"The real voyage of discovery consists not in seeking new landscapes but in having new eyes."*
>
> —Marcel Proust

_____

_____

_____

_____

_____

_____

_____

_____

"Patience and perseverance have a magical effect before which difficulties disappear and obstacles vanish."

–John Quincy Adams

_____

_____

_____

_____

_____

_____

_____

_____

_____

_____

_____

_____

_____

_____

_____

LOCK IT IN

_____

_____

_____

"Pleasure in the job
puts perfection in
the work."

–Aristotle

_____

_____

_____

_____

_____

_____

_____

_____

_____

_____

_____

_____

_____

_____

_____

_____

_____

_____

_____

_____

_____

_____

74

_____

_____

_____

_____

_____

_____

_____

_____

_____

_____

_____

_____

_____

_____

_____

_____

_____

_____

_____

_____

_____

_____

76

iCHANGE REPORT

_____

_____

_____

"Don't judge each day by the harvest you reap but by the seeds you plant."

–Robert Louis Stevenson

_____

_____

_____

_____

_____

_____

_____

_____

_____

_____

_____

_____

_____

_____

_____

_____

_____

_____

_____

Lab number: _____ Name of Lab: _____

GET REAL

_____
_____
_____
_____
_____
_____
_____
_____
_____
_____
_____
_____
_____
_____
_____
_____
_____
_____
_____
_____
_____
_____
_____
_____
_____

"It is not the critic who counts, nor the man who points out how the strong man stumbled, or where the doer of deeds could have done them better. The credit belongs to the man who is actually in the arena, whose face is marred by dust and sweat and blood; who strives valiantly; who errs and comes short again and again; who knows great enthusiasms, great devotions; who spends himself in a worthy cause; who, at the best, knows in the end the triumph of high achievement, and who, at the worst, if he fails, at least fails while daring greatly, so that his place shall never be with those timid souls who know neither victory nor defeat."

—Theodore Roosevelt

_____

_____

_____

_____

_____

_____

_____

_____

_____

_____

_____

_____

_____

_____

_____

_____

_____

_____

_____

_____

_____

_____

_____

_____

_____

> _"I have learned that if one advances confidently in the direction of his dreams, and endeavors to live the life he has imagined, he will meet with a success unexpected in common hours."_
>
> —Henry David Thoreau

81

*"Nothing endures
but change."*

—Heraclitus

GET READY

_____

_____

_____

_____

_____

_____

_____

_____

> *"There is nothing like returning to a place that remains unchanged to find the ways in which you yourself have altered."*
>
> —Nelson Mandela

_____

_____

_____

_____

_____

_____

_____

_____

_____

_____

_____

_____

_____

_____

_____

_____

_____

83

*"Life without a pur-
pose is a languid,
drifting thing; every
day we ought to re-
view our purpose,
saying to ourselves,
'This day let me
make a sound be-
ginning.'"*

—Thomas Kempis

_____

_____

_____

_____

_____

_____

_____

_____

_____

_____

_____

_____

_____

_____

_____

_____

_____

_____

_____

_____

_____

_____

_____

_____

_____

_____

_____

_____

"Know what's weird? Day by day, nothing seems to change, but pretty soon.... everything's different."

—Calvin from *Calvin and*

Hobbes

GET GOING

"If you don't like something, change it; if you can't change it, change the way you think about it."

—Mary Engelbreit

> *"The only differ-*
> *ence between a rut*
> *and a grave is their*
> *dimensions."*
>
> —Anonymous

_____
_____
_____
_____
_____
_____
_____
_____
_____
_____
_____
_____
_____
_____
_____
_____
_____
_____
_____
_____
_____
_____
_____
_____
_____
_____

_____

_____

_____

_____   *"Change yourself,*
                                                change your
_____   *fortunes."*

_____   —Portuguese Proverb

_____

_____

_____

_____

_____

_____

_____

_____   89

_____

_____

_____

_____

_____

_____

_____

_____

_____

_____

LOCK IT IN

"You must be the change you wish to see in the world."

—Mahatma Gandhi

"To keep our faces toward change and behave like free spirits in the presence of fate is strength undefeatable."

—Helen Keller

_____

_____

_____

_____

_____

"*Great spirits have always encountered violent opposition from mediocre minds.*"

—Albert Einstein

_____

_____

_____

_____

_____

_____

_____

93

_____

_____

_____

_____

_____

_____

_____

_____

_____

_____

_____

_____

iCHANGE REPORT

_____

_____

_____

_____

_____

_____

"Accept challenges, so that you may feel the exhilaration of victory."

—George S. Patton

_____

_____

_____

_____

_____

_____

_____

_____

_____

_____

_____

_____

_____

_____

GET REAL

"Challenges are what make life interesting; overcoming them is what makes life meaningful."

—Joshua J. Marine

"Difficulties are meant to rouse, not discourage. The human spirit is to grow strong by conflict."

—William Ellery Channing

GET READY

"We are like tea bags—we don't know our own strength until we're in hot water."

—Sister Busche

_____

_____

_____

_____

_____

_____

_____

"A smooth sea never made a skillful mariner."

—Anonymous

_____

_____

_____

_____

_____

_____

_____

_____

_____

_____

_____

_____

_____

_____

_____

> *"Count it all joy, my brethren, when you meet various trials, for you know that the testing of your faith produces steadfastness. And let steadfastness have its full effect, that you may be perfect and complete, lacking in nothing."*
>
> —James 1:24, RSV

GET GOING

> *"Nothing is impossible to a willing heart."*
>
> —John Heywood, sixteenth-century English poet

LOCK IT IN

*"Attitude deter-
mines altitude."*

—Anonymous

_____

_____

_____

_____

_____

_____

_____

_____

_____

_____

_____

_____

_____

_____

_____

_____

_____

_____

_____

_____

_____

_____

_____

_____

"Our deepest fear is not that we are inadequate. Our deepest fear is that we are powerful beyond measure. It is our light not our darkness that frightens us. Actually, who are you not to be? You are a child of God. Your playing small doesn't serve the world. There's nothing enlightened about shrinking so that other people won't feel insecure around you. We were born to make manifest the glory of God that is within us."

—Nelson Mandela, inaugural address, written by Marianne Williamson

"A ship is safe in harbor, but that's not what ships are for."

—William Shedd

iCHANGE REPORT

_____

_____

_____

_____

_____

_____

_____

_____

_____

"Many men go fishing all their lives not knowing it is not fish they are after."

—Henry David Thoreau

_____

_____

_____

_____

_____

_____

_____

_____

_____

_____

_____

_____

_____

_____

_____

_____

_____

_____

Lab number: _____ Name of Lab: _____

GET REAL

_____
_____
_____
_____
_____
_____
_____
_____
_____

"To understand the heart and mind of a person, look not at what he has already achieved, but at what he aspires to."

—Kahlil Gibran

_____
_____
_____
_____
_____
_____
_____
_____
_____
_____
_____
_____
_____
_____
_____
_____

*"There is nothing
either good or bad,
but thinking makes
it so."*

—William Shakespeare

"We have a choice every day regarding the attitude we will embrace for that day.... I am convinced that life is 10% what happens to me and 90% how I react to it. And so it is with you.... we are in charge of our attitudes."

—Charles Swindoll

GET READY

_____

_____

_____

_____

_____

_____

_____

_____

"A man sees in the world what he carries in his heart."

—Johann Wolfgang Goethe,

from "Faust"

_____

_____

_____

_____

_____

_____

_____

_____

_____

_____

_____

_____

_____

_____

_____

_____

_____

_____

*"No one can make
you feel inferior
without your
consent."*

—Eleanor Roosevelt

_____

_____

_____

_____

_____

_____

_____

_____

_____

"Ideals are like stars; you will not succeed in touching them with your hands, but like the seafaring man on the desert of waters, you choose them as your guides, and following them, you reach your destiny."

—Carl Schurz

_____

_____

_____

_____

_____

_____

_____

_____

_____

_____

_____

GET GOING

> *"Whether you think you can or think you can't—you are right."*
>
> —Henry Ford

> *"There are no guarantees. From the viewpoint of fear, none are strong enough. From the viewpoint of love, none are necessary."*
>
> —Emmanuel

_____

_____

_____

_____

_____

_____

_____

_____

_____

_____

_____

_____

_____

_____

_____

_____

_____

_____

_____

_____

_____

_____

_____

_____

_____

_____

"Seldom does an individual exceed his own expectations."

—Anonymous

LOCK IT IN

_____

_____

_____

_____

_____

"Security is a kind of death."

—Tennessee Williams,

Esquire, September, 1971

_____

_____

_____

_____

_____

_____

_____

_____

_____

_____

_____

_____

_____

_____

_____

_____

_____

_____

_____

"The only job where you start at the top, is digging a hole."

—Anonymous

_____

_____

_____

_____

_____

_____

_____

_____

> *"It is not our purpose to become each other; it is to recognize each other, to learn to see the other and honor him for what he is."*
>
> —Hermann Hesse

_____

_____

_____

_____

_____

_____

_____

_____

_____

_____

_____

_____

_____

_____

"Never giving up and pushing forward will unlock all the potential we are capable of."

—Christy Borgeld

iCHANGE REPORT

_____

_____

_____

_____

_____

> *"Now is the time.*
> *Needs are great,*
> *but your possibilities*
> *are greater."*
>
> —Bill Blackman

_____

_____

_____

_____

_____

_____

_____

129

_____

_____

_____

_____

_____

_____

_____

_____

_____

_____

_____

_____

_____

FREE WRITING SPACE

Free writing space. Journal on any topic of your choosing!

_____

_____

_____

_____

_____

_____

_____

_____

_____

_____

_____

_____

_____

_____

_____

_____

_____

_____

_____

_____

_____

_____

141

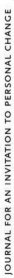